C000180583

The content contained within this bo
duplicated or transmitted without direct written permission
from the author or the publisher.
Under no circumstances will any blame or legal responsibility be
held against the publisher, or author, for any damages,
reparation, or monetary loss due to the information contained
within this book. Either directly or indirectly.

Legal Notice:

Disclaimer Notice:
Please note the information contained within this document is
for educational and entertainment purposes only. All effort has
been executed to present accurate, up to date, and reliable,
complete information. No warranties of any kind are declared or
implied. Readers acknowledge that the author is not engaging in
the rendering of legal, financial, medical or professional advice.
The content within this book has been derived from various
sources. Please consult a licensed professional before attempting
any techniques outlined in this book.
By reading this document, the reader agrees that under no
circumstances is the author responsible for any losses, direct or
indirect, which are incurred as a result of the use of information
contained within this document, including, but not limited to, —
errors, omissions, or inaccuracies.

TABLE OF CONTENTS

5

Fried Shrimp Po' Boy Sandwich Recipe

Prep Time: 20 minutes

Cook Time: 10 minutes

Total Time: 30 minutes

Ingredients

- 1 pound shrimp, deveined
- 1 teaspoon creole seasoning i used tony chachere
- 1/4 cup buttermilk
- 1/2 cup louisiana fish fry coating
- Cooking oil spray (if air frying) i use olive oil
- Canola or vegetable oil (if pan-frying) you will need enough oil to fill 2 inches of height in your frying pan.
- 4 french bread hoagie rolls i used 2 loaves, cut each in half 2 cups shredded iceberg lettuce
- 8 tomato slices
- Remoulade Sauce
- 1/2 cup mayo I used reduced-fat 1 tsp minced garlic
- 1/2 lemon juice of
- 1 tsp Worcestershire

My Lean & Green Recipes

A Collection of Lean & Green Air Fryer Recipes
for your Everyday Meals

Roxana Sutton

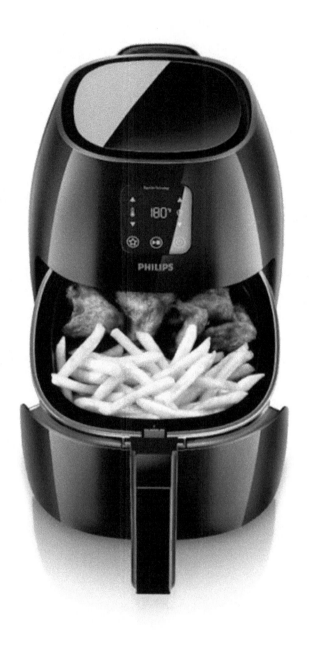

- 1/2 tsp Creole Seasoning I used Tony Chachere
- 1 tsp Dijon mustard
- 1 tsp hot sauce
- 1 green onion chopped

Instructions

Remoulade Sauce

Combine all of the ingredients in a small bowl. Refrigerate before serving while the shrimp cooks.

Shrimp And Breading

Marinate the shrimp in the Creole seasoning and buttermilk for 30 minutes. I like to use a sealable plastic bag to do this.

Add the fish fry to a bowl. Remove the shrimp from the bags and dip each into the fish fry. Add the Pan Fry Air Fryer shrimp to the air fryer basket.

Heat a frying pan with 2 inches of oil to 350 degrees. Use a thermometer to test the heat. Fry the shrimp on both sides for 3-4 minutes until crisp.

Remove the shrimp from the pan and drain the excess grease using paper towels.

Spray the air fryer basket with cooking oil. Add the shrimp to the air fryer basket. Spritz the shrimp with cooking oil.

Cook the shrimp for 5 minutes at 400 degrees. Open the basket and flip the shrimp to the other side. Cook for an additional 3-5 minutes or until crisp.

Assemble the Po Boy Spread the remoulade sauce on the French bread.

Add the sliced tomato and lettuce, and then the shrimp.

Nutritional Facts

Serving: 1serving | Calories: 437kcal | Carbohydrates: 55g | Protein: 24g | Fat: 12g

Easy Air Fryer Rotisserie Roasted Whole Chicken

Prep Time: 15 minutes

Cook Time: 55 minutes

Resting: 15 minutes

Total Time: 1 hour 25 minutes

Ingredients

- 1 4.5-5 pounds whole chicken
- 1/2 fresh lemon
- 1/4 whole onion
- 4 sprigs of fresh thyme
- 4 sprigs of fresh rosemary
- Olive oil spray
- 1 teaspoon ground thyme i like to use ground thyme in addition to fresh thyme for optimal flavor.
- 1 teaspoon onion powder
- 1 teaspoon garlic powder
- Kosher salt to taste be sure to use kosher salt.

Instructions

I purchased my whole chicken ready with the contents of the cavity removed. If your chicken still has the giblets inside of it, you will need to remove them before cooking.

Stuff 1/2 of fresh-cut lemon and 1/4 of a chopped onion inside the cavity of the chicken along with the fresh rosemary and thyme.

Make sure the chicken is completely dry on the outside. Pat dry with paper towels if necessary. A dry chicken will help it crisp in the air fryer with the olive oil.

Spray olive oil onto both sides of the chicken using an oil sprayer.

Sprinkle the seasonings throughout and onto both sides of the chicken. You may elect to only season the bottom side of the chicken at this step. Because you will need to flip the chicken during the air frying process, you will likely lose some of the seasonings at this stage. My preference is to season both sides initially, and then re-assess if more seasoning (usually salt is needed later).

Line the air fryer with parchment paper. This makes for easy cleanup. Load the chicken into the air fryer basket with the breast side down.

Air fry the chicken for 30 minutes at 330 degrees.

Open the air fryer and flip the chicken. I gripped the chicken cavity with tongs to flip.

Re-assess if more seasoning is needed on the breasts, legs, and wings. Add additional if necessary.

Air fry for an additional 20-25 minutes until the chicken reaches an internal temperature of 165 degrees. Use a meat thermometer.

This step is important. Place the meat thermometer in the thickest part of the chicken, which is typically the chicken thigh area. I like to test the breast too, just to ensure the entire chicken is fully cooked.

Remove the chicken from the air fryer basket and place it on a plate to rest for at least 15 minutes before cutting into the chicken. This will allow the moisture to redistribute throughout the chicken before you cut into it.

Nutrition Facts

Calories: 340kcal | Carbohydrates: 2g | Protein: 33g | Fat: 22g

Air Fryer Beef Taco Fried Egg Rolls

Prep Time: 15 minutes

Cook Time: 25 minutes

Total Time: 40 minutes

Servings: 8

Ingredients

- 1 pound ground beef
- 16 egg roll wrappers i used wing hing brand
- 1/2 cup chopped onion i used red onion.
- 2 garlic cloves minced
- 16 oz can diced tomatoes and chilies i used mexican rotel.
- 8 oz refried black beans i used fat-free and 1/2 of a 16oz can.
- 1 cup shredded mexican cheese
- 1/2 cup whole kernel corn i used frozen Cooking oil spray
- Homemade taco seasoning
- 1 tablespoon chili powder
- 1 teaspoon cumin
- 1 teaspoon smoked paprika Salt and pepper to taste

Instructions

Add the ground beef to a skillet on medium-high heat along with the salt, pepper, and taco seasoning. Cook until browned while breaking the beef into smaller chunks.

Once the meat has started to brown add the chopped onions and garlic. Cook until the onions become fragrant.

Add the diced tomatoes and chilis, Mexican cheese, beans, and corn. Stir to ensure the mixture is combined.

Lay the egg roll wrappers on a flat surface. Dip a cooking brush in water. Glaze each of the egg roll wrappers with the wet brush along the edges. This will soften the crust and make it easier to roll.

Load 2 tablespoons of the mixture into each of the wrappers. Do not overstuff. Depending on the brand of egg roll wrappers you use, you may need to double wrap the egg rolls.

Fold the wrappers diagonally to close. Press firmly on the area with the filling, cup it to secure it in place. Fold in the left and right sides as triangles. Fold the final layer over the top to close. Use the cooking brush to wet the area and secure it in place.

Spray the air fryer basket with cooking oil.

Load the egg rolls into the basket of the Air Fryer. Spray each egg roll with cooking oil.

Cook for 8 minutes at 400 degrees. Flip the egg rolls. Cook for an additional 4 minutes or until browned and crisp.

Nutrition Facts

Calories: 348kcal | Carbohydrates: 38g | Protein: 24g | Fat: 11g

Air Fryer Beef Taco Fried Egg Rolls

Prep Time: 15 minutes

Cook Time: 25 minutes

Total Time: 40 minutes

Servings: 8

Ingredients

- 1 pound ground beef
- 16 egg roll wrappers i used wing hing brand
- 1/2 cup chopped onion i used red onion.
- 2 garlic cloves minced
- 16 oz can diced tomatoes and chilies i used mexican rotel.
- 8 oz refried black beans i used fat-free and 1/2 of a 16oz can.
- 1 cup shredded mexican cheese
- 1/2 cup whole kernel corn i used frozen Cooking oil spray
- Homemade Taco Seasoning
- 1 tablespoon chili powder
- 1 teaspoon cumin
- 1 teaspoon smoked paprika

- Salt and pepper to taste

Instructions

Add the ground beef to a skillet on medium-high heat along with the salt, pepper, and taco seasoning. Cook until browned while breaking the beef into smaller chunks.

Once the meat has started to brown add the chopped onions and garlic. Cook until the onions become fragrant.

Add the diced tomatoes and chilis, Mexican cheese, beans, and corn. Stir to ensure the mixture is combined.

Lay the egg roll wrappers on a flat surface. Dip a cooking brush in water. Glaze each of the egg roll wrappers with the wet brush along the edges. This will soften the crust and make it easier to roll.

Load 2 tablespoons of the mixture into each of the wrappers. Do not overstuff. Depending on the brand of egg roll wrappers you use, you may need to double wrap the egg rolls.

Fold the wrappers diagonally to close. Press firmly on the area with the filling, cup it to secure it in place. Fold in the left and right sides as triangles. Fold the final layer over the top to close. Use the cooking brush to wet the area and secure it in place.

Spray the air fryer basket with cooking oil.

Load the egg rolls into the basket of the Air Fryer. Spray each egg roll with cooking oil.

Cook for 8 minutes at 400 degrees. Flip the egg rolls. Cook for an additional 4 minutes or until browned and crisp.

Nutrition Facts

Calories: 348kcal | Carbohydrates: 38g | Protein: 24g | Fat: 11g

Easy Crispy Garlic Parmesan Chicken Wings

Prep Time: 15 minutes

Cook Time: 45 minutes

Total Time:1 hour

Servings: 4

Ingredients

- 1 pound chicken wings (drummettes)
- 1/2 cup flour see recipe notes for low carb substitute.
- 1/2 cup grated parmesan divided into two 1/4 cup servings
- 1/2 tablespoon mccormicks grill mates chicken seasoning you can use your favorite chicken rub.
- Salt and pepper to taste
- Cooking oil i use olive oil.
- 3 garlic cloves minced
- 1 tablespoon butter
- 1 tablespoon olive oil

Instructions

Oven and Baking Instructions

Preheat the oven to 375 degrees.

Pat the chicken dry and place it on a large bowl or plastic bag.

Add the flour, 1/4 cup of grated parmesan, chicken seasoning, salt, and pepper to the chicken. Ensure the chicken is fully coated.

Line a sheet pan with parchment paper and add the wings. Spritz the chicken wings with cooking oil. Bake the wings for 20 minutes and then open and flip the wings. Spritz with cooking oil. Bake for an additional 10 minutes.

Heat a saucepan on medium-high heat. Add the butter, 1 tablespoon of olive oil, garlic, and 1/4 cup of grated parmesan.

Cook for 2-3 minutes until the butter and cheese have melted.

Remove the chicken from the oven and drizzle the wings in the garlic parmesan sauce. Return the chicken to the oven. Bake for an additional 10-15 minutes.

Garnish with parsley and parmesan if you wish.

Air Fryer Instructions

Pat the chicken dry and place it on a large bowl or plastic bag.

Add the flour, 1/4 cup of grated parmesan, chicken seasoning, salt, and pepper to the chicken. Ensure the chicken is fully coated.

Line the air fryer basket with air fryer parchment paper. Place the chicken on the parchment paper. Spritz the chicken with olive oil.

Air fry for 15 minutes at 400 degrees.

Open the air fryer and flip the chicken. Spritz the chicken with cooking oil. Cook for an additional 5 minutes.

Heat a saucepan on medium-high heat. Add the butter, 1 tablespoon of olive oil, garlic, and 1/4 cup of grated parmesan.

Cook for 2-3 minutes until the butter and cheese have melted.

Remove the chicken from the air fryer and drizzle it with the garlic parmesan butter. Return the chicken to the air fryer. Air fryer for an additional 3-4 minutes on 400 degrees. Garnish with parsley and parmesan if you wish.

Nutrition Facts

Calories: 374kcal | Carbohydrates: 11g | Protein: 26g | Fat: 24g

Air Fryer Crispy Crab Rangoon

Prep Time: 15 minutes

Cook Time: 15 minutes

Total Time: 30 minutes

Ingredients

- 4 or 6 oz cream cheese, softened If you prefer creamy crab rangoon use 6 oz
- 4 or 6 oz lump crab meat If you prefer your crab rangoon to have more cream cheese and less crab, use 4 oz. Seafood lovers may want to go for 6 oz
- 2 green onions, chopped
- 21 wonton wrappers
- 2 garlic cloves, minced
- 1 teaspoon Worcestershire sauce
- Salt and pepper to taste
- Cooking oil I use olive oil.

Instructions

You can soften your cream cheese by heating it in the microwave for 20 seconds.

Combine the cream cheese, green onions, crab meat, Worcestershire sauce, salt, pepper, and garlic in a small bowl. Stir to mix well.

Layout the wonton wrappers on a working surface. I used a large, bamboo cutting board. Moisten each of the wrappers with water. I use a cooking brush, and brush it along all of the edges.

Load about a teaspoon and a half of filling onto each wrapper. Be careful not to overfill.

Fold each wrapper diagonally across to form a triangle. From there bring up the two opposite corners toward each other. Don't close the wrapper yet. Bring up the other two opposite sides, pushing out any air. Squeeze each of the edges together. Be sure to check out the recipe video above for illustration.

Spritz the air fryer basket with cooking oil.

Load the crab rangoon into the air fryer basket. Do not stack or overfill. Cook in batches if needed. Spritz with oil.

Place the Air Fryer at 370 degrees. Cook for 10 minutes.

Open and flip the crab rangoon. Cook for an additional 2-5 minutes until they have reached your desired level of golden brown and crisp.

Remove the crab rangoon from the air fryer and serve with your desired dipping sauce.

Nutrition Facts

Calories: 98kcal | Carbohydrates: 12g | Protein: 7g | Fat: 3g

Air Fryer 3 Ingredient Fried Catfish

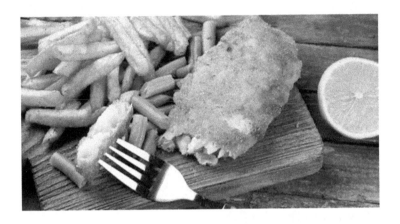

Prep Time5 minutes

Cook Time: 20 minutes

Total Time: 25 minutes

Ingredients

- 4 catfish fillets
- 1/4 cup Louisiana Fish Fry Coating
- 1 tbsp olive oil
- 1 tbsp chopped parsley optional

Instructions

Pat the catfish dry.

Sprinkle the fish fry onto both sides of each fillet. Ensure the entire filet is coated with seasoning. Spritz olive oil on the top of each filet.

Place the filet in the Air Fryer basket. Do not stack the fish and do not overcrowd the basket. Cook in batches if needed. Close and cook for 10 minutes at 400 degrees.

Open the air fryer and flip the fish. Cook for an additional 10 minutes. Open and flip the fish.

Cook for an additional 2-3 minutes or until desired crispness. Top with optional parsley.

Nutrition Facts

Calories: 208kcal | Carbohydrates: 8g | Protein: 17g | Fat: 9g

Air Fryer Bang Bang Fried Shrimp

Prep Time: 10 minutes

Cook Time: 20 minutes

Total Time: 30 minutes

Ingredients

- 1 pound raw shrimp peeled and deveined
- 1 egg white 3 tbsp
- 1/2 cup all-purpose flour
- 3/4 cup panko bread crumbs
- 1 tsp paprika
- Mccormick's grill mates montreal chicken seasoning to taste
- Salt and pepper to taste
- Cooking oil
- Bang Bang Sauce
- 1/3 cup plain, non-fat Greek yogurt
- 2 tbsp Sriracha
- 1/4 cup sweet chili sauce

Instructions

Preheat Air Fryer to 400 degrees. Season the shrimp with the seasonings.

Place the flour, egg whites, and panko bread crumbs in three separate bowls.

Create a cooking station. Dip the shrimp in the flour, then the egg whites, and the panko bread crumbs last.

When dipping the shrimp in the egg whites, you do not need to submerge the shrimp. Do a light dab so that most of the flour stays on the shrimp. You want the egg white to adhere to the panko crumbs.

Spray the shrimp with cooking oil.

Add the shrimp to the Air Fryer basket. Cook for 4 minutes.

Open the basket and flip the shrimp to the other side. Cook for an additional 4 minutes or until crisp.

Bang Bang Sauce

Combine all of the ingredients in a small bowl. Mix thoroughly to combine.

Nutrition Facts

Calories: 242kcal | Carbohydrates: 32g | Protein: 37g | Fat: 1g

Air Fryer Parmesan Truffle Oil Fries

Prep Time 10 minutes

Cook Time 40 minutes

Total Time 50 minutes

Ingredients

- 3 large russet potatoes peeled and cut lengthwise
- 2 tbsp white truffle oil
- 2 tbsp parmesan shredded
- 1 tsp paprika
- salt and pepper to taste
- 1 tbsp parsley chopped

Instructions

Place the sliced potatoes in a large bowl with cold water.

Allow the potatoes to soak in the water for at least 30 minutes, preferably an hour.

Spread the fries onto a flat surface and dry them completely with paper towels. Coat them with 1 tbsp of the white truffle oil and seasonings.

Add half of the fries to the Air Fryer basket. Adjust the temperature to 380 degrees and cook for 15-20 minutes. Set a timer for 10 minutes and stop and shake the basket at the 10-minute mark (once).

Use your judgment. If the fries need to be crisper, allow them to cook for additional time. If the fries look crisp before 15 minutes, remove them. I cooked both of my batches for almost 20 minutes.

When the first half finishes, cook the remaining half.

Add the remaining truffle oil and parmesan to the fries immediately upon removing them from the Air Fryer.

Top with shredded parsley. Serve!

Nutrition Facts

Calories: 233kcal

Air Fryer Low-Fat Weight Watchers Mozzarella Cheese Sticks

Prep Time: 10 minutes

Cook Time: 16 minutes

Total Time: 26 minutes

Ingredients

- 10 pieces mozzarella string cheese I used Weight Watchers Smoked Flavor
- 1 cup Italian breadcrumbs
- 1 egg
- 1/2 cup flour
- 1 cup marinara sauce
- Salt and pepper to taste

Instructions

Season the breadcrumbs with salt and pepper.

Create a workstation by adding the flour, bread crumbs, and eggs to separate bowls. Dip each string of cheese in flour, then egg, and last the breadcrumbs.

Freeze the sticks for one hour so that they harden. This will help the cheese maintain the stick shape while frying.

Season your Air Fryer basket before each use so that items do not stick. I like to glaze the basket with coconut oil using a cooking brush.

Turn the Air Fryer on 400 degrees. Add the sticks to the fryer.

Cook for 8 minutes. Remove the basket. Flip each stick. You can use tongs, but be careful not to manipulate the shape. I used my hands to flip them. They weren't too hot. Cook for an additional 8 minutes.

Allow the sticks to cool for 5 minutes before removing them from the pan. Some of the sticks may leak cheese on the outside. Allow the sticks to cool, and then use your hands to correct the shape.

Nutrition Facts

Calories: 224kcal | Carbohydrates: 19g | Protein: 17g | Fat: 7g

Air Fryer Carrots (Three Ways)

Prep Time: 5 minutes

Cook Time: 20 minutes

Total Time: 25 minutes

Ingredients

- 4 cups sliced carrots (1/4-inch thick), washed and patted dry
- 2 tablespoons extra virgin olive oil
- *Savory Version*
- 1/2 teaspoon garlic powder
- 1/2 teaspoon dried basil
- 1/2 teaspoon dried oregano
- 1/2 teaspoon dried parsley
- 1/2 teaspoon kosher salt
- 1/4 teaspoon ground black pepper
- *Sweet Version*
- 1 tablespoon coconut sugar
- 1/2 tablespoon maple syrup
- 1/4 teaspoon kosher salt
- 1/8 teaspoon crushed red pepper flakes

- *Spicy Version*
- 1 teaspoon ground cumin
- 1 teaspoon smoked paprika
- 1/2 teaspoon kosher salt
- 1/8 teaspoon cayenne pepper
- 1/8 teaspoon ground black pepper

Instructions

Add the sliced carrots to a large bowl and evenly coat with oil. Add your choice of seasonings and toss to coat.

Place carrots in the air fryer basket and air fry on 400F for 18-20 minutes, or until fork-tender. Shake or stir the carrots after about 10 minutes. Serve immediately.

Nutritional Facts

Total Fat: 7.3g Total Carbohydrate: 12.2g Sugar: 5.8g

Calcium: 45.9mg Sat Fat: 1.1g Sodium: 239.8mg Fiber: 3.6g

Protein: 1.3g Vitamin C: 7.3mg Iron: 0.5g

Air Fryer Butternut Squash (Home Fries)

Prep Time: 10 minutes

Cook Time: 20 minutes

Total Time: 30 minutes

Ingredients

- 4 cups chopped butternut squash, 1-inch cubes (see cutting tips above)
- 2 tablespoons extra virgin olive oil
- 1 tablespoon maple syrup
- 1 teaspoon dried oregano
- 1/2 teaspoon garlic powder
- 1/2 teaspoon smoked paprika
- 1/2 teaspoon kosher salt
- 1/4 teaspoon ground chipotle chili pepper
-

Instructions

In a large bowl, add the squash cubes along with the other ingredients. Toss until the cubes are well coated.

Arrange the cubes in a single layer in the air fryer basket and air fry on 400F for 15-20 minutes, or until the squash is fork-tender and a little crispy on the outside. Shake or stir the cubes at the mid-way point. Carefully remove from the air fryer and serve immediately.

Nutritional Facts

Calories: 140 Total Fat: 7.2g

Total Carbohydrate: 20.5g Sugar: 6.2g

Calcium: 81.2mg Sat Fat: 1g Sodium: 302.3mg Fiber: 3.2g Protein: 1.6g Vitamin C: 29.4mg Iron: 1.3g

Air Fryer Mushrooms

Prep Time: 5 minutes

Cook Time: 15 minutes

Ingredients

- 7 oz 200 grams chestnut mushrooms
- 2 tsp vegetable oil
- 2 tsp low sodium soy sauce or tamari sauce
- 1 sprig rosemary
- ½ tsp salt and pepper

Instructions

Cut the mushrooms into thick slices, I usually cut each into 2 halves but if it's too big then I cut into smaller pieces. Try to make the size of the slices even so everything cooks evenly.

In a white bowl, toss the mushrooms with the rest of the ingredients so everything is well coated in soy, oil, and seasonings.

No need to preheat the Air Fryer. Place the mushrooms directly into the Air Fryer basket, and cook at 356f (180) for about 15 minutes flipping halfway through.

Open the Air Fryer basket and check every 5 minutes, shake the basket and decide how much longer you would like to cook the mushrooms for.

The mushrooms should be cooked well, but not dried out or burnt. So make sure not to overcook them. Serve with some extra sea salt flakes, and red chili flakes if desired.

Nutrition

Calories: 30kcal | Carbohydrates: 2g | Protein: 1g | Fat: 2g | Saturated Fat: 1g | Sodium: 377mg | Potassium: 222mg | Fiber: 1g | Sugar: 1g | Calcium: 9mg | Iron: 1mg

Easy Air Fryer Baked Potatoes

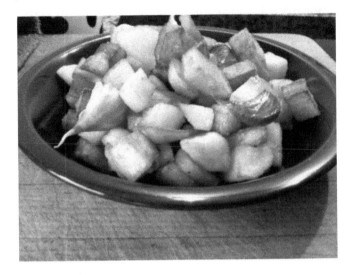

Prep Time: 5 minutes

Cook Time: 35 minutes

Total Time: 40 minutes

Ingredients

- 4 medium russet potatoes scrubbed and dried
- 4 teaspoons olive oil
- 1 teaspoon kosher sea salt plus more for serving if desired

Instructions

Preheat the air fryer to 375°F for about 10 minutes. Wash, dry, and prick each potato

Drizzle each potato with oil and sprinkle with salt.

Place 2 to 4 potatoes in your air fryer, depending on size.

Set air fryer to cook at 375° for 35 minutes, or until potatoes are fork-tender.

Use tongs to remove potatoes from the air fryer basket then carefully cut a slit in the top of each one. Add desired toppings & enjoy!

Nutrition

Serving: 1g | Calories: 204kcal | Carbohydrates: 38g | Protein: 5g | Fat: 4g | Saturated Fat: 1g | Sodium: 592mg | Potassium: 888mg | Fiber: 3g | Sugar: 1g | Vitamin C: 12mg | Calcium: 28mg | Iron: 2mg

Crispy Spicy Air Fryer Okra

Prep Time: 10 Minutes

Cook Time: 10 Minutes

Total Time: 20 Minutes

Ingredients

- 1 1/4 lb fresh okra

For the egg wash:

- 1 egg
- 1/2 tsp coriander
- 1/2 tsp smoked paprika
- 1/2 tsp chili powder (optional)
- Pinch of salt

For the panko breading:

- 1 cup gluten-free flaked panko breading
- 1 tsp coriander
- 1 tsp smoked paprika
- 1/2 tsp chili powder (optional)
- 1/2 tsp garlic powder
- 2 tbsp parsley

- 1/4 tsp each salt and pepper

Instructions

Rinse okra and dry thoroughly - I used paper towels to do so.

Prepare egg wash by mixing the egg with coriander, smoked paprika, chili powder (if using), and salt in a bowl.

Prepare to bread by mixing panko bread flakes with coriander, smoked paprika, chili powder (if using), garlic powder, parsley, salt, and pepper.

Then, using one hand, dip the dried okra in the spiced egg wash and drop it onto the plate with the breading.

Then, using the other hand, coat the okra well with the spiced panko breading. Repeat this with all the okra.

When the okra is all breaded, place them in a single layer at the bottom of your air fryer basket and spray them with your favorite cooking spray.

For best results, preheat the air fryer to 400 degrees for 2-3 minutes.

Set the air fryer to air fry the okra at 400 degrees for 4-5 minutes. Then open the air fryer, and using tongs, flip the okra over and air fry for 4-5 minutes at 400 degrees. Repeat if you have any more breaded okra (depending on the size of your air fryer, this might take 2- 3 batches to cook - but the result works it.

Enjoy with your favorite sauces!

Nutrition Information

Calories: 150 Total Fat: 3g Saturated Fat: 1g Trans Fat: 0g

Unsaturated Fat: 2g Cholesterol: 66mg Sodium: 302mg Carbohydrates: 23g Fiber: 4g

Sugar: 4g Protein: 8g

Air Fryer Radishes (Healthy Side Dish)

Prep Time: 10 minutes

Cook Time: 15 minutes

Total Time: 25 minutes

Ingredients

- 1 pound (or 454 gram packages) fresh radishes or about 3 cups halved
- 1 tablespoon extra virgin olive oil
- 1/2 teaspoon dried oregano
- 1/2 teaspoon kosher salt
- 1/4 teaspoon garlic powder
- 1/4 teaspoon onion powder
- Dash of ground black pepper

Instructions

Wash and trim the radishes, scrubbing off any dirt and cutting off any dark spots. Pat dry with a paper towel.

Slice the radishes in half so they are roughly 1-inch pieces (it doesn't need to be exact), or quarter them if they are larger.

Place the radishes in a large bowl and evenly coat with oil. Add the seasonings and toss to combine. Place radishes in the air fryer basket and air fry on 400F for 15-17 minutes, or until fork-tender. Shake or stir the radishes after about 10 minutes. Serve immediately.

Nutritional Facts

Calories: 48 Total Fat: 3.6g

Total Carbohydrate: 3.4g Sugar: 0g

Calcium: 33.7mg Sat Fat: 0.5g Sodium: 373.4mg Fiber: 1.7g Protein: 1.3g Vitamin C: 32.9mg Iron: 1mg

Air Fryer Zucchini And Onions

Total Time: 30 mins

Ingredients

- 2-3 zucchini small-medium sized
- 1 red onion
- 2 tbsp olive oil or avocado oil
- 1/2 tsp dried basil
- 1/2 tsp salt
- 1/2 tsp dried oregano
- 1/2 tsp garlic powder
- 1/4 tsp black pepper

Instructions

Do the Prep Work

Preheat your Air Fryer to 400F.

Meanwhile, wash and dice the zucchini and onions, at least twice the size of the holes in your air fryer basket.

In a bowl, toss the vegetables, oil, and all the Italian seasonings together. Cook the Dish

Pour the vegetable mixture into the heated air fryer, then shake or spread the vegetables so they're evenly spaced out in the basket. Close and set the timer for 20 minutes.

Halfway through cook time, open the air fryer and shake the basket or turn the vegetables with a spoon or spatula. Close and allow to finish cooking, then season to taste if needed and serve. Note: Sometime in the final two to three minutes, open the air fryer to make sure the vegetables aren't beginning to burn.

Nutrition

Calories: 91kcal | Carbohydrates: 6g | Protein: 2g | Fat: 7g | Saturated Fat: 1g | Sodium: 300mg | Potassium: 296mg | Fiber: 1g | Sugar: 4g | Vitamin A: 196IU | Vitamin C: 20mg | Calcium: 25mg | Iron: 1mg

Air Fryer Baby Potatoes (Easy Side Dish)

Prep Time: 5 minutes

Cook Time: 18 minutes

Total Time: 23 minutes

Ingredients

- 4 cups baby potatoes, skin on, pre-washed, and halved 1 lime, juiced
- 1 tablespoon extra virgin olive oil
- 1 tablespoon chili powder
- 1/2 teaspoon sea salt

Instructions

Place potatoes in a large bowl and coat them with lime juice. Drain any excess juice. Add the oil, chili powder, and sea salt and stir until potatoes are well coated.

Arrange the potatoes in a single layer in the air fryer basket. Roast on 400F for 15-18 minutes, or until the potatoes are tender with crispy edges. You can check on them after 7-8 minutes and give them a shake or stir.

Serve immediately (while hot and crispy).

Nutritional Facts

Calories: 95 Total Fat: 2.6g

Total Carbohydrate: 17g Sugar: 1.4g

Calcium: 14.6mg Sat Fat: 0.4g Sodium: 248.6mg Fiber: 1.7g Protein: 1.9g Vitamin C: 11.3mg Iron: 0.8mg

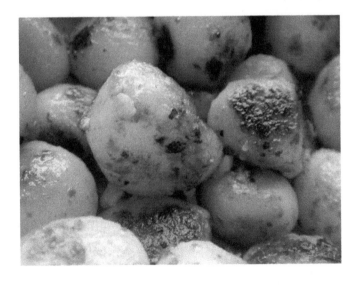

Air Fryer Broccoli Cheese Bites

Prep Time: 50 mins

Active Time: 20 mins

Total Time: 1 hr 10 mins

Ingredients

- 10 oz. fresh broccoli florets
- 1/4 cup water
- 1 large egg
- 1 1/2 cups shredded cheddar cheese
- 3/4 cup bread crumbs (panko or traditional)
- 1/2 tsp. kosher salt
- 1/2 tsp. black pepper

Instructions

Place broccoli and water in a microwave-safe container with a microwave-safe lid (if you don't have a lid you can use plastic wrap). Place lid lightly on top or cover tightly with plastic wrap. Microwave for 4 minutes.

Remove from microwave and allow to cool enough to handle. Chop very finely then place in a bowl. Add egg, cheese, bread crumbs, salt, and pepper to the broccoli and mix well. Grab a rimmed baking sheet.

Scoop out 1 1/2 tablespoons of the broccoli mixture and squeeze and form into a ball. Set on a baking sheet. Continue until you've used all the mixture. Place in the freezer for 30 minutes.

Place broccoli bites in an air fryer in a single layer and cook at 350 degrees F for 5-10 minutes depending on your air fryer. You may need to do this in batches (I did). Cover lightly with foil to keep warm while others are baking.

Nutritional Facts

Calories: 91kcal | Carbohydrates: 6g | Protein: 2g | Fat: 7g | Saturated Fat: 1g | Sodium: 300mg | Potassium: 296mg | Fiber: 1g | Sugar: 4g | Vitamin A: 196IU | Vitamin C: 20mg | Calcium: 25mg | Iron: 1mg

Healthy Air Fryer Eggplant [Oil Free]

Prep Time: 35 minutes

Cook Time: 15 minutes

Total Time: 50 minutes

Ingredients

- 1.5 lb eggplant cut into half-inch pieces (approx 1 medium-sized)
- 2 tbsp low sodium vegetable broth
- 1 tsp garlic powder
- 1 tsp paprika
- 1/2 tsp dried oregano
- 1/4 tsp dried thyme
- 1/4 tsp black pepper optional

Instructions

Wash and dice your eggplant into half-inch pieces. (See step by step photos above if needed.)

Now place your cut up eggplant in a large colander and place the colander inside a bowl. Generously sprinkle with salt and let it sit for 30 minutes. Then transfer to a clean, dry dishtowel, and using another dish towel, or paper towels, press and pat them dry.

Now, wipe out the bowl that was sitting under your colander and place the dry eggplant inside. Add the broth and all the seasoning to the bowl and mix well to evenly coat the pieces.

Place in your air fryer basket, set to 380 degrees, and cook for 15-20 minutes, tossing once at the halfway point. Cook until nicely golden, and fork-tender, then serve warm with a sprinkle of fresh parsley or chives and sriracha mayo for dipping.

Nutrition Facts

Calories: 48kcal | Carbohydrates: 11g | Protein: 2g | Fat: 1g | Saturated Fat: 1g | Sodium: 161mg | Potassium: 413mg | Fiber: 5g | Sugar: 6g | Vitamin A: 322IU | Vitamin C: 4mg | Calcium: 15mg | Iron: 1mg

How To Make Air Fryer Tortilla Chips (With Five Flavour Options!)

Prep Time: 10 minutes

Cook Time: 9 minutes

Total Time: 19 minutes

Ingredients

Salt And Vinegar

- 6 corn tortillas
- 1 tablespoon extra virgin olive oil
- 1/2 tablespoon white vinegar
- 1 teaspoon kosher salt

Zesty Cheese

- 6 corn tortillas
- 2 tablespoons extra virgin olive oil
- 2 teaspoons nutritional yeast
- 1/2 teaspoon smoked paprika
- 1/4 teaspoon kosher salt

Spicy Chipotle

- 6 corn tortillas
- 1 tablespoon extra virgin olive oil
- 1/2 teaspoon ground chipotle chili pepper

- 1/4 teaspoon kosher salt

Chili Lime

- 6 corn tortillas
- 1 tablespoon extra virgin olive oil
- 1/2 tablespoon lime juice
- 1 teaspoon chili powder
- 1/4 teaspoon kosher salt

Maple Cinnamon

- 6 corn tortillas
- 1 tablespoon extra virgin olive oil
- 1/2 tablespoon maple syrup
- 1/2 teaspoon ground cinnamon
- 1/2 teaspoon coconut suga

Instructions

In a small bowl, whisk together the oil with the ingredients for your flavor choice. Brush a light coating of the mixture on both sides of the tortillas.

Cut each tortilla into quarters to form triangles.

Arrange the tortilla triangles in a single layer in your air fryer basket. (You will need to do this in batches).

Air fry on 350F for about 7-9 minutes, or until they start to brown around the edges. (Note: the maple cinnamon chips will take 5-7 minutes).

Let the chips cool enough to handle and then transfer them to a wire rack to cool completely. They will get crunchier as they cool.

Store in an airtight container at room temperature and enjoy within 5 days.

Nutritional Facts

Calories: 156 Total Fat: 6g

Total Carbohydrate: 24g Sugar: 0g

Calcium: 91.6mg Sat Fat: 0.8g Sodium: 780.9mg Fiber: 2.7g Protein: 3g Vitamin C: 0mg Iron: 0.7mg

Air Fryer Asparagus

Prep Time: 5 minutes

Cook Time: 6 minutes

Total Time: 11 minutes

Ingredients

- 1 lb fresh asparagus (16 oz.)
- 2 tsp extra virgin olive oil
- Sea salt to taste

Instructions

Wash the asparagus spears and pat them dry. Trim the ends enough so that they fit in the air fryer basket (about 1 to 1 ½ inches up from the bottom).

Add the asparagus to a rectangular container with a tight-fitting lid or a zip-top bag along with the olive oil and salt. Shake until asparagus is well-coated.

If your air fryer has a separate elevated crisping tray or plate, be sure to insert it. Add the asparagus to the air fryer basket and air fry at 400° F for 6-9 minutes, shaking the basket every few minutes. Thinner spears will take less time to cook while thicker spears will take longer. Asparagus should be tender with a slight crisp. Add more sea salt to taste before serving, if desired.

Nutrition

Calories: 43kcal | Carbohydrates: 4g | Protein: 2g | Fat: 2g | Saturated Fat: 1g | Fiber: 2g

Air Fryer Pumpkin Fries

Prep Time: 15 minutes

Cook Time: 15 minutes

Total Time: 30 minutes

Ingredients

- 2 mini pumpkins, peeled, seeded, and cut into 1/2-inch slices (see cutting tips above)
- 2 teaspoons extra virgin olive oil
- 1/2 teaspoon garlic powder
- 1/2 teaspoon smoked paprika
- 1/2 teaspoon kosher salt

Instructions

Quicker version – air fry in one large batch:

Add the pumpkin slices to a large bowl and toss with oil and seasonings.

Place all the pumpkin in the air fryer basket and air fry on 400F for about 15 minutes, or until fork- tender. Shake or stir them at the mid-way point.

Nutritional Facts

Calories: 60 Total Fat: 2.5g

Total Carbohydrate: 10g Sugar: 4g

Calcium: 31.4mg Sat Fat: 0.4g Sodium: 156.9mg Fiber: 0.9g
Protein: 1.6g Vitamin C: 13.1mg Iron: 1.2mg

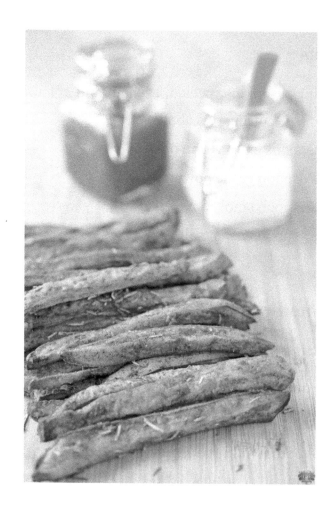

Lemon Garlic Air Fryer Roasted Potatoes

Prep Time: 10 Mins

Cook Time: 30 Mins

Air Fryer Preheating Time: 5 Mins

Total Time: 45 Mins

Ingredients

- 900 g / 2 lb potatoes (about 4 large ones)
- 2 tablespoons oil of choice, avocado, olive, vegetable, sunflower are all fine
- 1 teaspoon salt
- 1 teaspoon freshly ground black pepper
- 2 lemons
- 1 entire head of garlic
- 4 big (approx 4 inches long) fresh rosemary stems

Instructions

Peel the potatoes and cut them into large pieces.

With a large potato, I generally get 5 pieces.

Put the cut potatoes in a bowl and cover with cold water. Leave to soak for 15 minutes, then drain and pour the potatoes onto a clean dish towel. Bundle it up around them and rub them dry.

Dry the bowl you had them in and return them, then pour in the oil and sprinkle in the salt and pepper. Stir to coat them all evenly.

Preheat your Air Fryer if it has a preheat function, then add the potatoes carefully to the hot basket and cook on 350°F (175 °C) for 15 minutes.

While they are cooking, break up the head of garlic into individual cloves and remove any skin that is loose and papery. Leave the rest of the skin intact.

Cut the 2 lemons in half lengthways. Save one half for juicing, then cut the other halves into 3 wedges each.

Once the 15 minutes is up, open the Air Fryer and squeeze the juice from the half of lemon over the potatoes. Throw in the garlic cloves and the lemon wedges and give it all a really good toss together. Tuck in the rosemary stalks amongst the potatoes.

Return the basket to the Air Fryer and cook for a further 15 minutes. Check. They should be done, but if you prefer them a little more golden, put them back on for 5 minutes.

Pick out the woody rosemary sticks and serve the potatoes with the garlic cloves and the lemon wedges. Guests can squeeze the soft, sweet cloves of garlic out of their skins and eat it with the potatoes and the caramelized lemon.

To serve

When serving be sure to get some of the roasted garlic cloves and lemon wedges in each portion, then while eating, smush the caramelized lemon against the potatoes, squeeze that sweet roasted garlic out of its papery skin and eat it all together. And that's your potato game changed FOREVER!

Nutrition

Calories: 172kcal Carbohydrates: 28g Protein: 5g

Fat: 6g

Saturated Fat: 1g Sodium: 485mg Potassium: 817mg Fiber: 6g

Sugar: 1g Vitamin A: 23IU Vitamin C: 44mg Calcium: 72mg Iron: 6mg

Air Fryer Broccoli

Prep Time: 5 minutes

Cook Time: 15 minutes

Total Time: 20 minutes

Ingredients

- 1 pound (450 grams) broccoli cut into florets
- 1 tablespoon olive oil
- ½ teaspoon salt
- ¼ teaspoon ground black pepper
- ¼ teaspoon chili flakes optional

Instructions

Wash the broccoli head, and cut it into florets.

In a mixing bowl, toss the broccoli florets with olive oil, salt, pepper, and chili flakes.

Add to the Air Fryer basket, and cook at 390°F (200°C) for 15 minutes flipping at least twice while cooking.

Serve with lemon wedges.

Nutrition

Calories: 70kcal | Carbohydrates: 8g | Protein: 3g | Fat: 4g | Saturated Fat: 1g | Sodium: 330mg | Potassium: 358mg | Fiber: 3g | Sugar: 2g | Vitamin A: 744IU | Vitamin C: 101mg | Calcium:

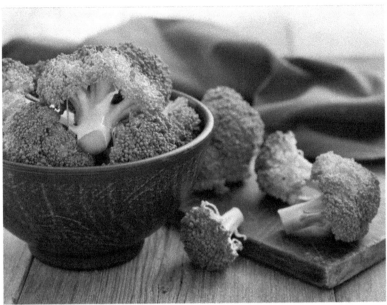

53mg | Iron: 1mg

Air Fryer Cauliflower

Prep Time: 8 mins

Cook Time: 12 mins

Total Time: 20 mins

Ingredients

- 1 head cauliflower
- 2 tbsp olive oil
- 1 tsp salt
- 2 tsp onion powder
- To Top: lime wedge and parmesan

Instructions

Cut your cauliflower into florets.

Toss the cauliflower in olive oil, salt, and onion salt.

Add the cauliflower into the air fryer basket (try to have it in a single layer if possible, cook in two batches if too many overlap).

Cook for 12-15 minutes on 375F.

When done, serve with parmesan shaved on top and some lime squeezed on top.

Nutrition

Serving: 4servings | Calories: 102kcal | Carbohydrates: 8g | Protein: 3g | Fat: 7g | Saturated Fat: 1g | Sodium: 626mg | Potassium: 442mg | Fiber: 3g | Sugar: 3g | Vitamin C: 70mg | Calcium: 36mg | Iron: 1mg

Air Fryer Tater Tots

Prep Time: 15 mins

Cook Time: 20 mins

Total Time: 35 mins

Ingredients

- 6 large potatoes or 8 medium, peeled
- 2 tbsp corn starch (cornflour)
- 1 1/2 tsp dried oregano
- 1 tsp garlic powder
- Salt

Instructions

Preheat the air fryer to 350 F / 180C.

Boil the potatoes till they are about half cooked and then plunge them into a cold water bath to stop the cooking process and cool them down.

Using a box shredder, shred the cooled potatoes into a large bowl, then squeeze out any excess water. Add in the rest of the ingredients and combine. Then form the mixture into individual tater tots (I was able to make about 20).

Place half of the homemade tater tots into the air fryer basket (making sure they don't touch) and cook for 18-20 minutes till golden brown. Turn the tots twice during cooking so that they brown evenly.

Remove the tater tots and keep warm, then repeat steps to make the remaining air fryer tater tots. Serve your air fryer tater tots with a side of vegan ranch dressing or tomato sauce for dipping.

Nutrition

Calories: 204kcal | Carbohydrates: 44g | Protein: 8g | Sodium: 32mg | Potassium: 1328mg | Fiber: 8g | Vitamin C: 36.4mg | Calcium: 102mg | Iron: 10.5mg

Air Fryer Beets (Easy Roasted Beets)

Prep Time: 10 minutes
Cook Time: 20 minutes
Total Time: 30 minutes

Ingredients

- 3 cups fresh beets, peeled and cut into 1-inch pieces (see note)
- 1 tablespoon extra virgin olive oil
- 1/2 teaspoon kosher salt
- Pinch of ground black pepper

Instructions

Add the beets, oil, salt, and pepper to a large bowl and toss to combine.

Place the beets in the air fryer basket and air fry on 400F for 18-20 minutes, or until fork-tender. Stir or shake them a few times while air frying.

Nutritional Facts

Calories: 74 Total Fat: 3.7g Total Carbohydrate: 9.8g Sugar: 6.9g

Calcium: 16.6mg Sat Fat: 0.5g Sodium: 234.mg Fiber: 2.9g
Protein: 1.6g Vitamin C: 5mg Iron: 0.8mg

Crispy Air Fryer Brussels Sprouts

Prep Time: 5 mins

Cook Time: 10 mins

Total Time: 15 mins

Ingredients

- 340 grams Brussels sprouts
- 1-2 tbsp olive oil
- Salt, to taste Pepper, to taste
- Garlic powder, to taste

Instructions

Trim and half your Brussels sprouts and lightly coat them with olive oil. Coat with a mixture of salt, pepper, and garlic powder.

Place the Brussels sprouts in the air fryer at 350F for 10 minutes. Shaking the basket once or twice during the cooking time.

Serve immediately or warm.

Nutritional Value

Calories: 91kcal | Carbohydrates: 6g | Protein: 2g | Fat: 7g | Saturated Fat: 1g | Sodium: 300mg | Potassium: 296mg | Fiber:

1g | Sugar: 4g | Vitamin A: 196IU | Vitamin C: 20mg | Calcium: 25mg | Iron: 1mg

Air-Fried Cauliflower With Almonds And Parmesan

Prep: 10 mins

Cook: 15 mins

Total: 25 mins

Servings: 4

Ingredients

- 3 cups cauliflower florets
- 3 teaspoons vegetable oil, divided
- 1 clove garlic, minced
- ⅓ cup finely shredded Parmesan cheese
- ¼ cup chopped almonds
- ¼ cup panko bread crumbs
- ½ teaspoon dried thyme, crushed

Instructions

Place cauliflower florets, 2 teaspoons oil, and garlic in a medium bowl; toss to coat. Place in a single layer in an air fryer basket.

Cook in the air fryer at 360 degrees F (180 degrees C), for 10 minutes, shaking the basket halfway through.

Return cauliflower to the bowl and toss with the remaining 1 teaspoon oil. Add Parmesan cheese, almonds, bread crumbs, and thyme; toss to coat. Return cauliflower mixture to the air fryer basket and cook until mixture is crisp and browned about 5 minutes.

Nutrition Facts

Calories: 148; Protein 6.7g; Carbohydrates 11g; Fat 10.1g; Cholesterol 5.9mg; Sodium 157.7mg.

Air Fryer Falafel

Prep Time: 20 mins

Cook: 20 mins

Additional: 1 day

Total: 1 day

Ingredients

- 1 cup dry garbanzo beans
- 1 ½ cups fresh cilantro, stems removed
- ¾ cup fresh flat-leafed parsley stems removed
- 1 small red onion, quartered
- 1 clove garlic
- 2 tablespoons chickpea flour
- 1 tablespoon ground coriander
- 1 tablespoon ground cumin
- 1 tablespoon sriracha sauce
- salt and ground black pepper to taste
- ½ teaspoon baking powder
- ¼ teaspoon baking soda cooking spray

Instructions

Soak chickpeas in a large amount of cool water for 24 hours. Rub the soaked chickpeas with your fingers to help loosen and remove skins. Rinse and drain well. Spread chickpeas on a large clean dish towel to dry. Blend chickpeas, cilantro, parsley, onion, and garlic in a food processor until rough paste forms. Transfer mixture to a large bowl. Add chickpea flour, coriander, cumin, sriracha, salt, and pepper and mix well. Cover bowl and let the mixture rest for 1 hour.

Preheat an air fryer to 375 degrees F (190 degrees C). Add baking powder and baking soda to the chickpea mixture. Mix using your hands until just combined. Form 15 equal-sized balls and press slightly to form patties. Spray falafel patties with cooking spray.

Place 7 falafel patties in the preheated air fryer and cook for 10 minutes. Transfer cooked falafel to a plate and repeat with the remaining 8 falafel, cooking for 10 to 12 minutes.

Nutrition Facts

Calories: 60; Protein 3.1g; Carbohydrates 9.9g; Fat 1.1g; Sodium 97.9mg.

Air-Fried Carrots With Balsamic Glaze

Prep Time: 10 mins

Cook Time: 10 mins

Total Time: 20 mins

Ingredients

- Olive oil for brushing
- 1 tablespoon olive oil
- 1 teaspoon honey
- ¼ teaspoon kosher salt
- ¼ teaspoon ground black pepper
- 1 pound tri-colored baby carrots
- 1 tablespoon balsamic glaze
- 1 tablespoon butter
- 2 teaspoons chopped fresh chives

Instructions

Brush an air fryer basket with olive oil.

Whisk together 1 tablespoon olive oil, honey, salt, and pepper in a large bowl. Add carrots and toss to coat. Place carrots in the air fryer basket in a single layer, in batches, if needed.

Cook in the air fryer at 390 degrees F (200 degrees C), stirring once, until tender, about 10 minutes. Transfer warm cooked carrots to a large bowl, add balsamic glaze and butter and toss to coat. Sprinkle with chives and serve.

Nutrition Facts

Calories: 117; Protein 0.8g; Carbohydrates 11.9g; Fat 7.7g; Cholesterol 7.6mg; Sodium 228mg.

Simple Air Fryer Brussels Sprouts

Prep Time: 5 mins

Cook Time: 30 mins

Total Time: 35 mins

Ingredients

- 1 ½ pound Brussels sprouts
- 2 tablespoons olive oil
- 1 teaspoon garlic powder
- 1 teaspoon salt
- ½ teaspoon ground black pepper

Instructions

Preheat the air fryer to 390 degrees F (200 degrees C) for 15 minutes.

Place Brussels sprouts, olive oil, garlic powder, salt, and pepper in a bowl and mix well. Spread evenly in the air fryer basket. Cook for 15 minutes, shaking the basket halfway through the cycle.

Nutrition Facts

Calories: 91; Protein 3.9g; Carbohydrates 10.6g; Fat 4.8g; Sodium 416.2mg.

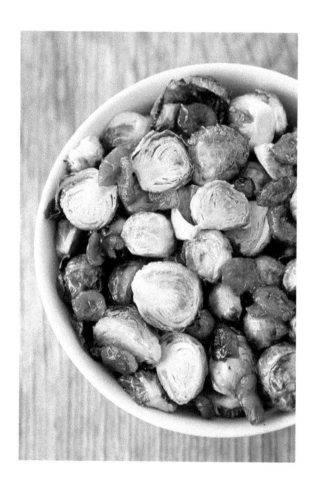

Air Fryer Potato Wedges

Prep Time: 5 mins

Cook Time: 30 mins

Total Time: 35 mins

Ingredients

- 2 medium Russet potatoes, cut into wedges
- 1 ½ tablespoon olive oil
- ½ teaspoon paprika
- ½ teaspoon parsley flakes
- ½ teaspoon chili powder
- ½ teaspoon sea salt
- ⅛ teaspoon ground black pepper

Instructions

Preheat air fryer to 400 degrees F (200 degrees C).

Place potato wedges in a large bowl. Add olive oil, paprika, parsley, chili, salt, and pepper, and mix well to combine.

Place 8 wedges in the basket of the air fryer and cook for 10 minutes.

Flip wedges with tongs and cook for an additional 5 minutes. Repeat with the remaining 8 wedges.

Nutrition Facts

Calories: 129; Protein 2.3g; Carbohydrates 19g; Fat 5.3g; Sodium 230.2mg.

Air-Fryer Roasted Veggies

Prep Time: 20 mins

Cook Time: 10 mins

Total Time: 30 mins

Ingredients

- ½ cup diced zucchini
- ½ cup diced summer squash
- ½ cup diced mushrooms
- ½ cup diced cauliflower
- ½ cup diced asparagus
- ½ cup diced sweet red pepper
- 2 teaspoons vegetable oil
- ¼ teaspoon salt
- ¼ teaspoon ground black pepper
- 1/4 teaspoon seasoning, or more to taste

Instructions

Preheat the air fryer to 360 degrees F (180 degrees C).

Add vegetables, oil, salt, pepper, and desired seasoning to a bowl. Toss to coat; arrange in the fryer basket.

Cook vegetables for 10 minutes, stirring after 5 minutes.

Nutrition Facts

Calories:37; Protein 1.4g; Carbohydrates 3.4g; Fat 2.4g; Sodium 152.2mg.

Air Fryer Roasted Asparagus

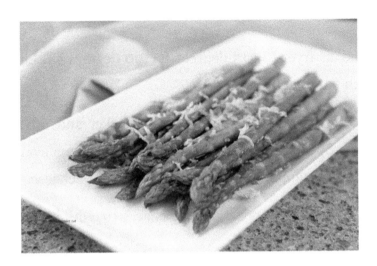

Prep Time: 10 mins

Cook Time: 10 mins

Total Time: 20 mins

Ingredients

- 1 bunch fresh asparagus, trimmed Avocado oil cooking spray
- ½ teaspoon garlic powder
- ½ teaspoon himalayan pink salt
- ¼ teaspoon ground multi-colored peppercorns
- ¼ teaspoon red pepper flakes

- ¼ cup freshly grated parmesan cheese

Instructions

Preheat the air fryer to 375 degrees F (190 degrees C). Line the basket with parchment paper.

Place asparagus spears in the air fryer basket and mist with avocado oil. Sprinkle with garlic powder, pink Himalayan salt, pepper, and red pepper flakes. Top with Parmesan cheese.

Air fry until asparagus spears start to char, 7 to 9 minutes.

Nutrition Facts

Calories: 94; Protein 9g; Carbohydrates 10.1g; Fat 3.3g; Cholesterol 8.8mg; Sodium 739.2mg.

Air Fryer Sweet And Spicy Roasted Carrots

Prep Time: 5 mins

Cook Time: 20 mins

Total: 25 mins

Ingredients

- 1 serving cooking spray
- 1 tablespoon butter, melted
- 1 tablespoon hot honey (such as Mike's Hot Honey®)
- 1 teaspoon grated orange zest
- ½ teaspoon ground cardamom
- ½ pound baby carrots
- 1 tablespoon freshly squeezed orange juice
- 1 pinch salt and ground black pepper to taste

Instructions

Preheat an air fryer to 400 degrees F (200 degrees C). Spray the basket with nonstick cooking spray. Combine butter, honey, orange zest, and cardamom in a bowl. Remove 1 tablespoon of the sauce to a separate bowl and set aside. Add carrots to the remaining sauce and toss until all are well coated. Transfer carrots to the air fryer basket.

Air fry until carrots are roasted and fork-tender, tossing every 7 minutes, for 15 to 22 minutes. Mix orange juice with reserved honey-butter sauce. Toss with carrots until well combined. Season with salt and pepper.

Nutrition Facts

Calories: 129; Protein 0.9g; Carbohydrates 19.3g; Fat 6.1g; Cholesterol 15.3mg; Sodium 206.4mg.

Air Fryer One-Bite Roasted Potatoes

Prep Time: 5 mins

Cook Time: 10 mins

Total Time: 15 mins

Ingredients

- ½ Pound mini potatoes
- 2 teaspoons extra-virgin olive oil
- 2 teaspoons dry italian-style salad dressing mix
- Salt and ground black pepper to taste

Instructions

Preheat the air fryer to 400 degrees F (200 degrees C).

Wash and dry potatoes. Trim edges to make a flat surface on both ends.

Combine extra-virgin olive oil and salad dressing mix in a large bowl. Add potatoes and toss until potatoes are well coated. Place in a single layer into the air fryer basket. Cook in batches if necessary. Air fry until potatoes are golden brown, 5 to 7 minutes. Flip potatoes and air fry for an additional 2 to 3 minutes. Season with salt and pepper.

Nutrition Facts

Calories: 132; Protein 2.3g; Carbohydrates 20.3g; Fat 4.8g; Sodium 166.8mg.

Air Fryer Cauliflower Tots

Prep Time: 5 mins

Cook Time: 10 mins

Total Time: 15 mins

Ingredients

- 1 serving nonstick cooking spray
- 1 (16 ounces) package frozen cauliflower tots (such as Green Giant® Cauliflower Veggie Tots)

Instructions

Preheat air fryer to 400 degrees F (200 degrees C). Spray the air fryer basket with nonstick cooking spray.

Place as many cauliflower tots in the basket as you can, making sure they do not touch, cooking in batches if necessary.

Cook in the preheated air fryer for 6 minutes. Pull the basket out, turn tots over, and cook until browned and cooked through, about 3 minutes more.

Nutrition Facts

Calories: 147; Protein 2.7g; Carbohydrates 20g; Fat 6.1g; Sodium 493.6mg.

Air Fryer Sweet Potato Tots

Prep Time: 15 mins

Cook Time: 35 mins

Additional Time: 10 mins

Total Time: 1 hr

Ingredients

- 2 sweet potatoes, peeled
- ½ teaspoon cajun seasoning
- Olive oil cooking spray
- Sea salt to taste

Instructions

Bring a pot of water to a boil and add sweet potatoes. Boil until potatoes can be pierced with a fork but are still firm for about 15 minutes. Do not over-boil, or they will be messy to grate. Drain and let cool. Grate sweet potatoes into a bowl using a box grater. Carefully mix in Cajun seasoning. Form mixture into tot-shaped cylinders.

Spray the air fryer basket with olive oil spray. Place tots in the basket in a single row without touching each other or the sides of the basket. Spray tots with olive oil spray and sprinkle with sea salt.

Heat air fryer to 400 degrees F (200 degrees C) and cook tots for 8 minutes. Turn, spray with more olive oil spray, and sprinkle with more sea salt. Cook for 8 minutes more.

Nutrition Facts

Calories: 21; Protein 0.4g; Carbohydrates 4.8g; Sodium 36.2mg.

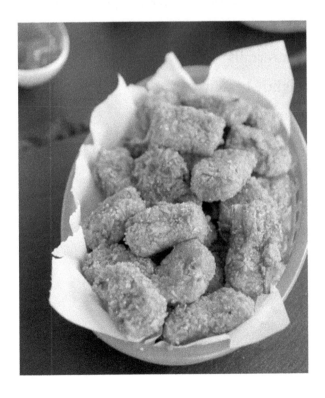

Air Fryer Fried Green Tomatoes

Prep Time: 15 mins

Cook Time: 20 mins

Total Time: 35 mins

Ingredients

- 2 green tomatoes, cut into 1/4-inch slices
- Salt and freshly ground black pepper to taste
- ⅓ cup all-purpose flour
- ½ cup buttermilk
- 2 eggs, lightly beaten
- 1 cup plain panko bread crumbs
- 1 cup yellow cornmeal
- 1 teaspoon garlic powder
- ½ teaspoon paprika
- 1 tablespoon olive oil, or as needed

Instructions

Season tomato slices with salt and pepper.

Set up a breading station in 3 shallow dishes: pour flour into the first dish; stir together buttermilk and eggs in the second dish; and mix breadcrumbs, cornmeal, garlic powder, and paprika in the third dish. Dredge tomato slices in flour, shaking off the excess. Dip tomatoes into the egg mixture, and then into the bread crumb mixture, making sure to coat both sides.

Preheat the air fryer to 400 degrees F (200 degrees C). Brush the fryer basket with olive oil. Place breaded tomato slices in the fryer basket, making sure they do not touch each other; cook in batches if necessary. Brush the tops of tomatoes with olive oil.

Cook for 12 minutes, then flip the tomatoes and brush again with olive oil. Cook until crisp and golden brown, 3 to 5 minutes more. Remove tomatoes to a paper towel-lined rack to keep crisp. Repeat with the remaining tomatoes.

Nutrition Facts

Calories: 219; Protein 7.6g; Carbohydrates 39.6g; Fat 5.3g; Cholesterol 62.8mg; Sodium 165.9mg.

Air Fryer Latkes

Prep Time: 20 mins

Cook Time: 20 mins

Total Time: 40 mins

Ingredients

- 1 (16 ounces) package frozen shredded hash brown potatoes, thawed
- ½ cup shredded onion 1 egg
- Kosher salt and ground black pepper to taste
- 2 tablespoons matzo meal
- Avocado oil cooking spray

Instructions

Preheat an air fryer to 375 degrees F (190 degrees C) according to the manufacturer's instructions. Layout a sheet of parchment or waxed paper.

Place thawed potatoes and shredded onion on several layers of paper towels. Cover with more paper towels and press to squeeze out most of the liquid.

Whisk together egg, salt, and pepper in a large bowl. Stir in potatoes and onion with a fork. Sprinkle matzo meal on top and stir until ingredients are evenly distributed. Use your hands to form the mixture into ten 3- to 4-inch wide patties. Place patties on the parchment or waxed paper.

Spray the air fryer basket with cooking spray. Carefully place half of the patties in the basket and spray generously with cooking spray.

Air-fry until crispy and dark golden brown on the outside, 10 to 12 minutes. (Check for doneness at 8 minutes if you prefer a softer latke.) Remove latkes to a plate. Repeat with remaining patties, spraying them with cooking spray before cooking.

Nutrition Facts

Calories: 97; Protein 3.3g; Carbohydrates 18.6g; Fat 6.5g; Cholesterol 32.7mg; Sodium 121.3mg.

Air Fryer Truffle Fries

Prep Time: 10 mins

Cook Time: 20 mins

Additional Time: 30 mins

Total Time: 1 hr

Ingredients

- 1 ¾ pounds russet potatoes, peeled and cut into fries
- 2 tablespoons truffle-infused olive oil
- ½ teaspoon paprika
- 1 tablespoon grated Parmesan cheese
- 2 teaspoons chopped fresh parsley
- 1 teaspoon black truffle sea salt

Instructions

Place fries in a bowl. Cover with water and let soak for 30 minutes. Drain and pat dry.

Preheat the air fryer to 400 degrees F (200 degrees C) according to the manufacturer's instructions. Place drained fries into a large bowl. Add truffle olive oil and paprika; stir until evenly combined. Transfer fries to the air fryer basket.

Air fry for 20 minutes, shaking every 5 minutes. Transfer fries to a bowl. Add Parmesan cheese, parsley, and truffle salt. Toss to coat.

Nutrition Facts

Calories: 226; Protein 4.8g; Carbohydrates 36.1g; Fat 7.6g; Cholesterol 1.1mg; Sodium 552mg.

Air Fryer Spaghetti Squash

Prep Time: 5 mins

Cook Time: 25 mins

Total Time: 30 mins

Ingredients

- 1 (3 pounds) spaghetti squash
- 1 teaspoon olive oil
- ¼ teaspoon sea salt
- ⅛ teaspoon ground black pepper
- ⅛ teaspoon smoked paprika

Instructions

Using a sharp knife, make a dotted line lengthwise around the entire squash. Place whole squash in the microwave and cook on full power for 5 minutes. Transfer to a cutting board and cut the squash in half lengthwise, using the dotted line as a guide. Wrap one half in plastic wrap and refrigerate for another use.

Spoon pulp and seeds out of the remaining half and discard. Brush olive oil over all of the flesh and sprinkle with salt, pepper, and paprika.

Preheat an air fryer to 360 degrees F (180 degrees C). Place spaghetti squash half skin-side-down in the basket. Cook for 20 minutes.

Transfer to a dish and fluff with a fork to create 'noodles'.

Nutrition Facts

Calories: 223; Protein 4.4g; Carbohydrates 47.2g; Fat 6.3g; Sodium 335.9mg.

Air Fryer Roasted Brussels Sprouts With Maple-Mustard Mayo

Prep Time: 5 mins

Cook Time: 10 mins

Total Time: 15 mins

Ingredients

- 2 tablespoons maple syrup, divided
- 1 tablespoon olive oil
- ¼ teaspoon kosher salt
- ¼ teaspoon ground black pepper
- 1 pound Brussels sprouts, trimmed and halved
- ⅓ cup mayonnaise
- 1 tablespoon stone-ground mustard

Instructions

Preheat the air fryer to 400 degrees F (200 degrees C).

Whisk together 1 tablespoon maple syrup, olive oil, salt, and pepper in a large bowl. Add Brussels sprouts and toss to coat. Arrange Brussels sprouts in a single layer in an air fryer basket without overcrowding; work in batches, if necessary. Cook for 4 minutes. Shake basket and cook until sprouts are deep golden brown and tender, 4 to 6 minutes more.

Meanwhile, whisk together mayonnaise, remaining 1 tablespoon maple syrup, and mustard in a small bowl. Toss sprouts in some of the sauce mixtures and/or serve as a dipping sauce.

Nutrition Facts

Calories: 240; Protein 4g; Carbohydrates 18.3g; Fat 18.3g; Cholesterol 7mg; Sodium 298mg.

Air Fryer Peri Peri Fries

Prep Time: 10 mins

Cook Time: 25 mins

Additional Time: 15 mins

Total Time: 50 mins

Ingredients

- 2 pounds russet potatoes
- ¼ teaspoon smoked paprika
- ¼ teaspoon chile powder
- ¼ teaspoon garlic granules
- ⅛ teaspoon ground white pepper
- ½ teaspoon salt
- 2 tablespoons grapeseed oil

Instructions

Peel and cut potatoes into 3/8-inch slices. Place into a bowl of water for 15 minutes to remove most of the starch. Transfer onto a clean kitchen towel and dry.

Preheat the air fryer to 350 degrees F (180 degrees C) for 5 minutes.

Mix paprika, chile powder, garlic. white pepper, and salt together in a small bowl.

Place the potatoes into a medium bowl and add grapeseed oil; mix well. Pour into the air fryer basket. Air fry for 10 minutes, shaking occasionally. Increase the temperature to 400 degrees F (200 degrees C) and air fry until golden brown, 12 to 15 more minutes.

Pour fries into a bowl, sprinkle with the seasoning mix, and shake the bowl to ensure fries are evenly covered. Taste and adjust salt, if necessary. Serve immediately.

Nutrition Facts

Calories: 237; Protein 4.7g; Carbohydrates 40g; Fat 7.1g; Sodium 304.4mg.

Air Fryer Fish And Chips

Prep Time: 20 mins

Cook Time: 30 mins

Additional Time: 1 hr 10 mins

Total Time: 2 hrs

Ingredients

Chips:

- 1 russet potato
- 2 teaspoons vegetable oil
- 1 pinch salt and ground black pepper to taste

Fish:

- ¾ cup all-purpose flour
- 2 tablespoons cornstarch
- ½ teaspoon salt
- ½ teaspoon garlic powder
- ¼ teaspoon baking soda
- ¼ teaspoon baking powder
- ¾ cup malt beer
- 4 (3 ounces) fillets cod fillets

Instructions

Peel the russet potato and cut it into 12 wedges. Pour 3 cups water into a medium bowl and submerge potato wedges for 15 minutes. Drain off water and replace it with fresh water. Soak wedges for 15 more minutes.

Meanwhile, mix flour, cornstarch, salt, garlic powder, baking soda, and baking powder in a bowl. Pour in 1/2 cup malt beer and stir to combine. If batter seems too thick, add remaining beer 1 tablespoon at a time.

Place cod fillets on a rimmed baking sheet lined with a drip rack. Spoon 1/2 of the batter over the fillets. Place rack in the freezer to allow the batter to solidify, about 35 minutes. Flip fillets over and coat the remaining side with the batter. Return to the freezer for an additional 35 minutes.

Preheat the air fryer to 400 degrees F (200 degrees C) for 8 minutes. Cook frozen fish fillets for 15 minutes, flipping at the halfway point.

Meanwhile, drain off water from potato wedges and blot dry with a paper towel. Toss with oil, salt, and pepper. Air fry for 15 minutes.

Nutrition Facts

Calories: 465; Protein 37.5g; Carbohydrates 62.3g; Fat 6.2g; Cholesterol 62.3mg; Sodium 1006mg.

"Everything" Seasoning Air Fryer Asparagus

Prep Time: 5 mins

Cook Time: 5 mins

Total Time: 10 mins

Ingredients

- 1 pound thin asparagus
- 1 tablespoon olive oil
- 1 tablespoon everything bagel seasoning
- 1 pinch salt to taste
- 4 wedge (blank)s lemon wedges

Instructions

Rinse and trim asparagus, cutting off any woody ends. Place asparagus on a plate and drizzle with olive oil. Toss with bagel seasoning until evenly combined. Place asparagus in the air fryer basket in a single layer. Work in batches if needed.

Heat the air fryer to 390 degrees F (200 degrees C).

Air fry until slightly soft, tossing with tongs halfway through, 5 to 6 minutes. Taste and season with salt if needed. Serve with lemon wedges.

Nutrition Facts

Calories: 70; Protein 2.7g; Carbohydrates 5.8g; Fat 3.6g; Sodium 281.5mg.

Air Fryer Tajin Sweet Potato Fries

Prep Time: 10 mins

Cook Time: 10 mins

Total Time: 20 mins

Ingredients

- Cooking spray
- 2 medium sweet potatoes, cut into 1/2-inch-thick fries
- 3 teaspoons avocado oil
- 1 ½ teaspoon chili-lime seasoning (such as tajin)

Dipping Sauce:

- ¼ cup mayonnaise
- 1 tablespoon freshly squeezed lime juice
- 1 teaspoon chili-lime seasoning (such as Tajin®) 4 lime wedges

Instructions

Preheat the air fryer to 400 degrees F (200 degrees C) for 5 minutes. Lightly spray the fryer basket with cooking spray.

Place sweet potato fries in a large bowl, drizzle with avocado oil, and stir. Sprinkle with 1 1/2 teaspoons chili-lime seasoning and toss well. Transfer to the air fryer basket, working in batches if necessary.

Cook sweet potato fries until brown and crispy, 8 to 9 minutes, shaking and turning the fries after 4 minutes.

While sweet potatoes are cooking, whisk together mayonnaise, lime juice, and chili-lime seasoning for the dipping sauce in a small bowl. Serve sweet potato fries with dipping sauce and lime wedges.

Nutrition Facts

Calories: 233; Protein 2g; Carbohydrates 24.1g; Fat 14.8g; Cholesterol 5.2mg; Sodium 390.1mg.

Air Fryer Fingerling Potatoes

Prep Time: 10 mins
Cook Time: 15 mins
Total Time: 25 mins

Ingredient

- 1 pound fingerling potatoes, halved lengthwise
- 1 tablespoon olive oil
- ½ teaspoon ground paprika
- ½ teaspoon parsley flakes
- ½ teaspoon garlic powder
- Salt and ground black pepper to taste

Instructions

Preheat an air fryer to 400 degrees F (200 degrees C).

Place potato halves in a large bowl. Add olive oil, paprika, parsley, garlic powder, salt, and pepper and stir until evenly coated.

Place potatoes in the basket of the preheated air fryer and cook for 10 minutes. Stir and cook until desired crispness is reached, about 5 more minutes.

Nutrition Facts

Calories: 120; Protein 2.4g; Carbohydrates 20.3g; Fat 3.5g; Sodium 46.5mg.

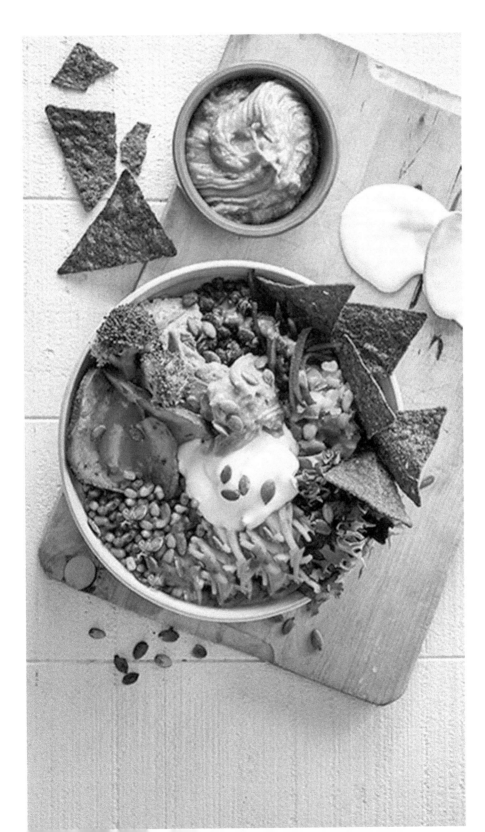

Lightning Source UK Ltd.
Milton Keynes UK
UKHW020645300421
382900UK00010B/326